Dedicated with Love,

to two special heroes of CHD -

My parents Ginny and Dick Putnam.

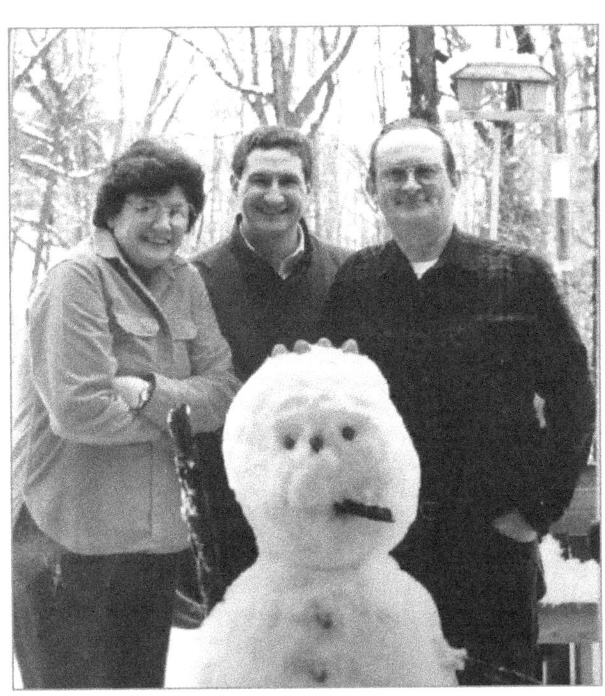

My Cardiac Trailblazers
Challenges and Blessings of My Journey with Congenital Heart Disease

Forward

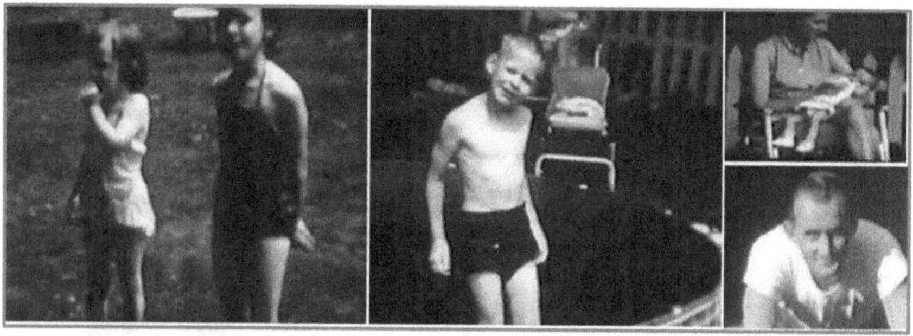

My name is Mike Putnam. I have no actual memory of that summer back in 1962. At about nine months of age, how could I? I wasn't old enough to walk, form ideas or express my thoughts. Fortunately, I do have a small, wonderful glimpse into my world at that time through a 2 minute and 20 second home movie clip filmed by my parents, Richard and Virginia Putnam. That clip, though short, reveals a great deal about me. It gives me a real sense of what would drive me and what would turn out to be most important to me throughout my life.

In the movie clip, I see my siblings, Kathy, age 6, Dick Jr., 5 and Carol, 3, happily splashing in a wading pool and playing on a swing-set in the backyard of our home at 29 Bixby Street in Bainbridge, New York.

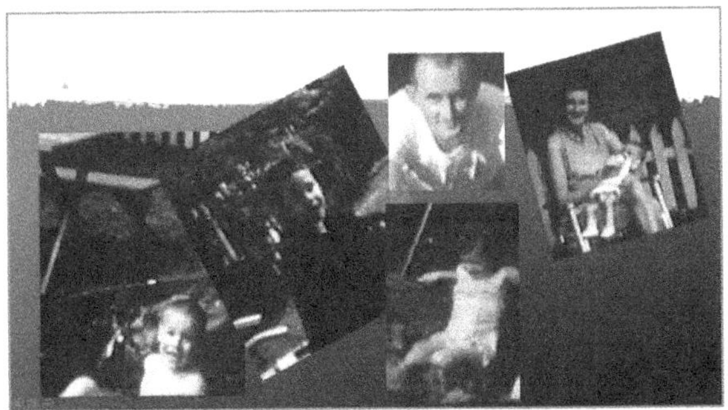

It's a warm sunny day with a gentle breeze blowing through the trees. The scene is picture-perfect, right down to the bright green grass and the white picket fence framing our backyard. In the background, my mother is sitting in a lawn chair, feeding me a bottle. A quick look from a distance supports this happy scene and conveys a sense that all is well with the Putnam family.

As Dad zooms in for a closer look, my attention is quickly drawn to something that is not quite right.   Close observation reveals clear evidence that my recently detected Congenital Heart Disease is quickly robbing me of my vitality.

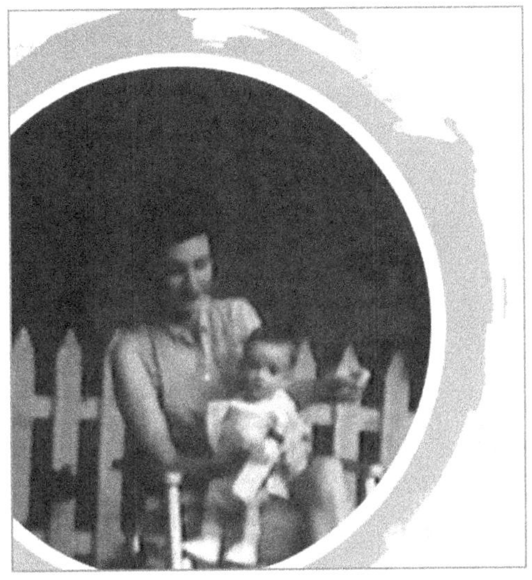

I see a pencil-thin pair of legs and a distinct look of fatigue. The diagnosis of double inlet left ventricle and a transposition of the great vessels was causing me to quickly lose weight and energy. My outlook was bleak.

A close-up shot of my face speaks very clearly to me in many ways. It's an expression I instantly recognize as one I've worn several times over my fifty-eight years. I look restless and clearly tired. Still, I am concentrating on the family activities going on around me. What really speaks to me is the slight frown, furrowed brow and determined expression that says, "I will get through this!"

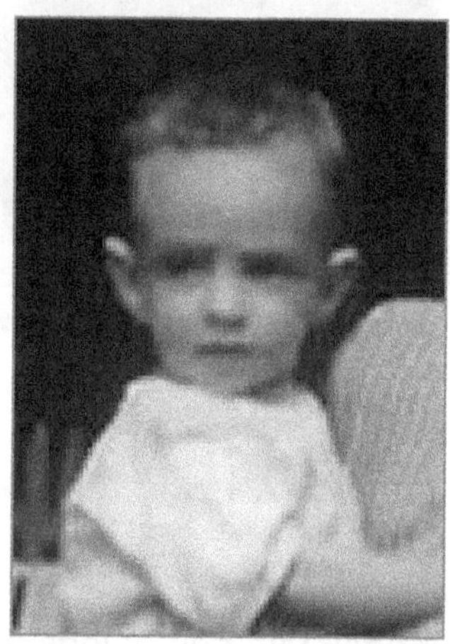

And so, it was in the Summer of 1962 for a 9-month-old boy with Congenital Heart Disease, facing a high-risk open-heart surgery as his one chance at survival. And so, it was for my parents, Ginny and Dick Putnam. They had to shoulder the entire load of uncertainty while searching for a way for me to survive. They were hoping for at least a few more years to give me a chance to be a part of this loving family and to enjoy some of those wonderful family memories captured on that 2 minute and

20 second movie clip. And so, it was for my siblings. They would come to understand the need take up for me whenever required. They would give me piggy-back rides when I was tired, pull me up the hill on a sled so I could enjoy a ride down or let me tag along with their friends, even when I could not keep up.

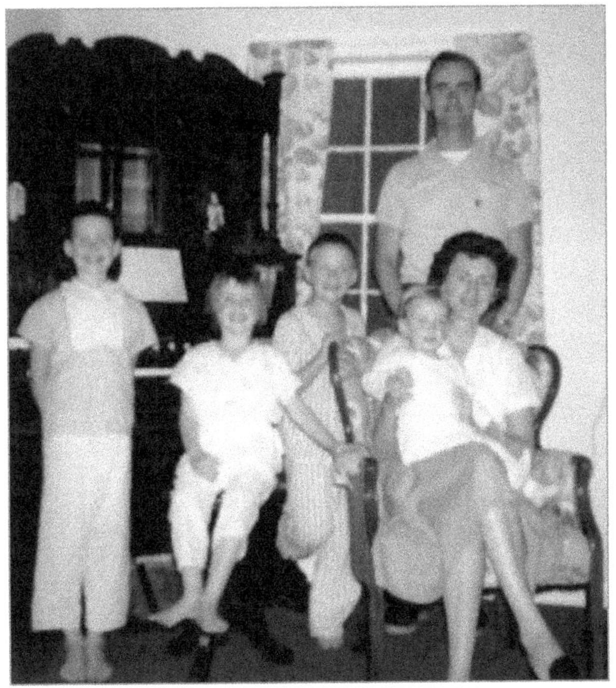

My Cardiac Trailblazers

Yes, my family members are the everyday heroes of my CHD journey even to this day. Necessity formed a great family team that summer in 1962. I did my part by surviving and thriving. They did theirs by making the right health decisions, supporting me at every step, and spoiling me a little. In return, they always expected me to uphold my responsibilities to be a full and active family member. True to my expression in the movie clip, I was up for that challenge!

My Cardiac Trailblazers

Challenges and Blessings of My Journey
with
Congenital Heart Disease

1 – *The Journey Begins*

In September 2018, I was reminded that it had been thirty years since my most recent open-heart surgery, a modified Fontan procedure, to address a quickly deteriorating situation due to underlying congenital heart disease (CHD). This milestone caused me to reflect on my journey with CHD. For the first time ever, I decided to take a holistic view of this eventful journey that has led me to where I am today at age 57. One of the challenges I faced as I started to think about my CHD journey was the realization that fifty-seven years is a long time. There is a great deal to be remembered, much more that has been forgotten and many peaks and valleys along the way.

Revisiting this 57-year journey reaffirmed for me a set of core beliefs that have carried me this far. I have strong faith in God, guiding me on a path through all the uncertainty facing a CHD baby, born in 1961 with L-transposition of the great vessels with ventricular septal defect (i.e. double inlet, left ventricle or single ventricle). God has blessed me with a wonderful, loving wife, Theresa and two incredible daughters, Ashley and Rachel. They along with my parents, Dick and Ginny and siblings, Kathy, Dick Jr. and Carol have been there with me, without exception, providing critical support every step of the way.

I have an unwavering confidence in the medical professionals known to me as my "Cardiac Trailblazers," who not only made it possible for me to survive but to

My Cardiac Trailblazers

thrive through their great care and cutting-edge open-heart surgeries in 1962, 1977 and 1988. Much of this is a result of the awe-inspiring talents of some of the best doctors in the world and the amazing achievements that have been made over the past six decades. It's clear to me that I've been blessed to be in the right situation with the right doctors, ready with leading medical solutions to allow me to live a fulfilling life. As a tribute to their collective talents, I was inspired to name our annual Congenital Heart Walk team (now numbering over 30 friends and family) the Cardiac Trailblazers '62.

Also clear to me is my will to persevere through the numerous challenges at long odds resulting in me being here to tell my story today. I'm comfortable with the belief that it is better, smarter and ultimately more powerful to trust in all these factors. My faith in God, medical science, my family and the human spirit resulted in me being here

My Cardiac Trailblazers

today. With that glimpse into my philosophy, here is a look at my CHD journey.

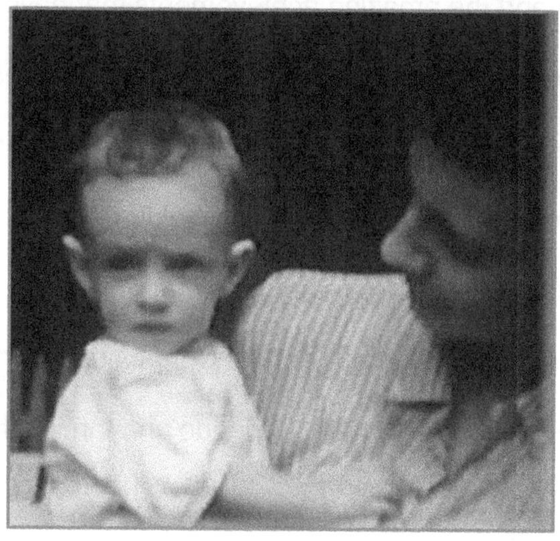

Figure 1 Summer 1962

2 - *New York, New York*

A few months after my birth in October 1961, it became apparent to my parents that something was not right. I wasn't thriving. This was soon confirmed by the local town doctor who indicated that I had a complex congenital heart defect. His grim prognosis provided my parents little hope that I would survive more than a few more months. Mom and Dad weren't convinced and decided to search elsewhere for help.

My parents' unwillingness to give up and a guiding hand eventually led us to a small regional hospital in Cooperstown, NY and through the doctors' connections, ultimately to Columbia Presbyterian Hospital in New York City. It was there that Dr. Sylvia Griffiths provided us with hope. Following an examination and tests, she recommended a relatively new surgical procedure known as pulmonary artery banding. If successful, it could mitigate many of the immediate dangers of my CHD and give me a fighting chance to live for about three to five years. The technique had been done successfully on older patients for several years, though not often on children less than two years of age.

With my condition rapidly deteriorating and no other options, my parents made the decision to have the doctors perform this new open-heart surgery. The procedure took place in October 1962 when I was just eleven months old. Given my small size and the surgical limitations of the day, this was a highly risky undertaking. I can't imagine how Mom and Dad must have felt sitting in the waiting room for the doctors to report the outcome, but I am certainly glad that I was not aware of any of it!

By all accounts, the surgery was a resounding success! I'm told the biggest post-surgical challenge was to keep me calm enough so that all the tubes and monitors would stay in place. I would simply not sit still. This increased activity level indicated I must have been feeling better very quickly after the surgery. I had an outstanding recovery and photos of me taken two months later, on Christmas 1962 show that I was alert, active and gaining weight. I looked like a normal, healthy toddler. I had a second chance and was ready to embrace it.

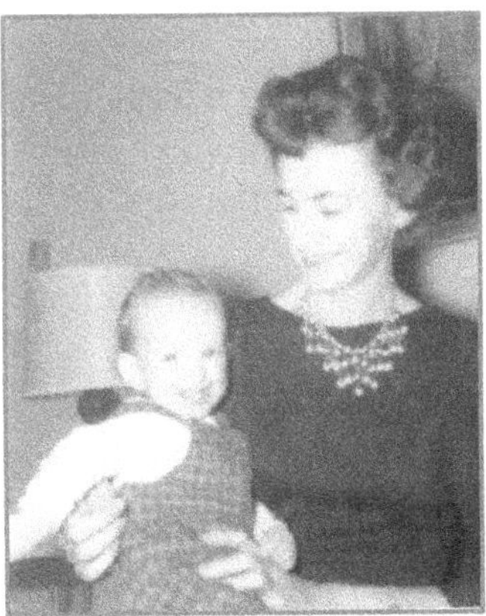

Figure 2 Christmas 1962

3 – *Blessings Abound*

In fact, for the next several years, I thrived and went about life as a normal child as much as possible. I was relatively healthy and as active as I could be until June 1968. At that time, I had a sudden bout with possible rheumatic fever. I remember my parents rushing me to the Cooperstown Hospital with our car on the verge of breaking down, but somehow the car didn't give out until we got to the hospital parking lot. It turned out, we had gotten there just in time for the doctors to prevent any permanent damage and I was effectively treated and eventually released after spending about a week in the hospital. To come through this potentially dangerous illness unharmed was another blessing.

On February 9, 1969, my parents drove me back to see Dr. Griffiths for a follow-up catheterization. On that day we unknowingly drove into one of the epic Nor'easters to hit New York in the 20th Century. The closer we got to New York, the harder it snowed, eventually causing Dad to pull the car off the road to clear the snow-packed windshield.   The car had gone too far into the snowbank and we found ourselves stuck. Dad's attempts to push us out with Mom driving appeared futile and it looked like we were going to be stranded there for the duration. Caught in the midst of the "Lindsay Snowstorm," blamed for killing 42 people stuck on the highways that day, we were again clearly in grave danger.

Dad tried once more to get us out and, in a miracle, Mom later attributed to angels lifting us up, the car seemed to effortlessly glide out of the snowbank and back onto the road. To this day I still get chills up my spine when I remember the smooth movement of the car back onto the highway, leading us safely to our destination.   No doctors or medical science were on hand to save us that day, but we were again the beneficiaries of a major blessing.

The results of that follow-up catheterization in 1969 were better than we could have hoped. There was no apparent damage from rheumatic fever and the pulmonary artery banding was working very well. The prognosis of a three to five-year lifespan had already exceeded seven years and I was doing fine. Dr. Griffiths' focus shifted to helping me live within my limitations. I began to understand those limitations, but I was always willing to push them as far as I could.

My unstated, but natural objective was simple: Be a normal kid. I would play as hard as I could and rest when I had to. I would do what I could to either keep up with the other kids or attempt to compensate in some way, while at the same time drawing the least attention to my limitations. Sometimes it worked, other times it didn't.

My Cardiac Trailblazers

My memories of that time between 1969 and 1977 are probably very similar to those of many kids. Aside from dealing with the heartbreak of being restricted from organized sports, I fit in well with my peers at school. I enjoyed most subjects, participated in gym class until high school and routinely engaged in neighborhood pick-up games after school.

I have countless fond memories of Kathy, Dick and Carol spending a lot of time with me and making sure I was included in ball games, sledding, skiing or Kick the Can. Kathy is six years older than I, Dick five and Carol three and so they must have dreaded their obligation at times, especially when they wanted to hang around with their friends and swap teenage stories. They never seemed to complain about it.

They each took very good care of me as I made my way through elementary school with very little thought to my CHD. One day there was Dick thrashing the two bullies who opened-up a big gash in my forehead after throwing rocks at me. Later in the day, Dick would feel the wrath of the bullies' older brother, but he didn't tell me that happened until years later. Another time, Kathy had to untangle me from choking on a rope that got caught around my neck while playing cowboy in the basement. I remember that incident really scaring Mom.

The ultimate rescue was when Carol saved me from certain drowning after I fell through the melting ice covering the creek that ran through our neighborhood. I still remember the enveloping darkness when going completely under water before splashing back to the surface in a panic and wailing for help. Carol was there in a flash and quickly pulled me up onto the dam to safety. She somehow got me home and back into dry clothes with no one knowing – a story we kept from my parents for

roughly 40 years. You might say I'm extremely fortunate to

have this protective family and a few close friends who

always seemed to be watching out for me!

4 – Most fun ... biggest challenge

After moving to Ohio in 1972, I was again blessed to be referred to another great pediatric cardiologist, Dr. Donald Hosier at Children's Hospital in Columbus. Dr. Hosier picked up the torch from Dr. Griffiths and impressed my parents with his calm, logical approach. He provided great care, understood that I could thrive by limiting myself and continued to give us confidence that he would be there for us when needed.

During this time, we also had the good fortune to move into a great neighborhood in Granville where I developed some close friendships. My neighborhood friends and I were always engaged in some activity throughout our middle school years and well into high school. Whether it was pick-up whiffle ball, football, basketball, ping-pong, or any other game, I could especially count on Jim Keller, Dave Marttala and Brad Bostian to include me in every activity while not making an issue of my limitations. For this, I'll always be grateful.

Things began to deteriorate quickly though in 1977 when I hit a teenage growth spurt my freshman year of high school. My growth was quickly outpacing the capacity for my pulmonary artery banding to allow enough oxygenated blood to circulate through my body. While I had been somewhat cyanotic with bluish fingertips growing up, it became severe as I grew during the first half of 1977. My exercise tolerance decreased rapidly as my body tried to grow. I quickly became frustrated by the reality that neighborhood football and whiffle ball games were no longer possible for me.

My world was closing in around me. I had an unhealthy look with my bluish skin color now noticeable to all. I endured "good natured teasing" from numerous kids at school which hurt more than I would admit. To cope, I withdrew as much as I could from most activities and avoided everyone except my family. Fortunately, my family and close friends stood by me and helped me endure this trying time.

The only time I felt alright physically was when I first woke up in the morning. That time each day provided me a fleeting moment of optimism until being reminded that simply getting ready for school was now a strenuous effort. The optimism faded as I forced myself through each day, dreading how the other kids in school were viewing me and struggling with the overwhelming fatigue that came with my situation.

A catheterization ordered by Dr. Hosier during that summer confirmed that I would need to have open-heart surgery to increase pulmonary blood flow and alleviate the symptoms. My body was determined to grow, but my anatomy would need some help to supply more oxygen to it. As my sophomore year of high school began, Mom had to drive me to and from the bus stop each day because I could no longer walk the quarter mile between there and our house. This time period was the most difficult of my life.

Fortunately, my parents and Dr. Hosier were guiding me in the right direction by scheduling surgery for October 1977. They knew very well that I needed to have surgery to survive, but I was in denial. I'm not sure my parents fully understood at the time that I was not coping with the reality at all.

I had a poor attitude as the surgery date approached. The denial continued and only came to a head as I was undergoing the final pre-surgery tests at Children's Hospital. I recall how I resented being treated like a child and not getting all the information, but I wasn't mature enough to listen to full disclosure either.

At that point, the assigned Resident on duty showed up in my room and proceeded to clinically explain all the risks of the upcoming Right Blalock-Taussig shunt procedure. His explanation included a small potential of losing use of my arm and possible amputation. As he coldly explained the risk of death during the procedure, I snapped! I slammed my fist down on the table, smashing the model I had been assembling, and ultimately created such a disruption that I was discharged from the hospital that day and sent home.

Dad and Mom must have been at their wit's end, trying to think of ways to get me to rethink my position. This was new territory for them. This time, they weren't making decisions for a toddler or a six-year-old with little input. They were dealing with a frightened sixteen-year-old who needed to both understand and come to terms with the required path forward.

My parents then made three brilliant decisions that changed the trajectory of the entire situation. The first decision was to consult my trusted Aunt Joan. Aunt Joan Dean and her husband Uncle Dizzy were doctors, both of whom I trusted implicitly growing up. Aunt Joan must have sensed that I felt cornered; everyone pushing me in a direction I did not want to go. She knew that a more subtle approach was needed to reopen my mind. She immediately voiced full support for me and the decision that I had forced in leaving the hospital. She told my parents that if I didn't feel good with the situation, I was right to not go through with it at that time.

Once I was calmer and I felt I had an ally, Aunt Joan put things in better perspective by explaining that the surgery would soon be over and it would allow me to be active again. Of course, my parents had told me the same things many times before but hearing it from Aunt Joan somehow made a difference.

The next decision was to place a phone call to Dr. Griffiths. My parents knew how much she had helped us in years past and that a conversation with her could really help all of us.   I don't remember any details of that phone call or what we discussed about the surgery. I'm not sure I was listening to her words at all. But I do remember just hearing her voice put me at ease and gave me confidence that I could get through this challenge.   I'm sure there were many other patients who have the same high regard for Dr. Griffiths as I do. I recently noticed a posting about her describing how she continues to stay involved by working in the Columbia Hospital one day per week even in her mid-nineties. She is an amazing doctor!

Decision three was also a great idea. It was to arrange a meeting with Dr. James W. Kilman, the surgeon assigned to my case. Dr. Kilman explained to me that while he was not a betting man, he would certainly bet on me in this situation. Dr. Kilman answered all my questions about the surgery, really taking the mystery out of what was to come and counteracting the Resident's stark assessment.

My parents' three-tiered strategy combined with Dr. Hosier's suggestion that the surgery take place at Ohio State University Hospital so that I would feel more like an adult worked well. It also provided a new venue away from the still fresh, unpleasant memories. I had what I needed

to comprehend and support the surgery with an open

mind. I just needed to get past my personal denial.

At the same time, the realities of my urgent need

for surgery were finally registering with me. Following my

hospital meltdown, I returned to the same bad situation at

school. The first week back I was upholding my

commitments by keeping statistics for the Granville High

School football team on a cold night in late October. I

remember having a very hard time even staying warm and

just walking the sideline to record the plays completely

wore me out. At the end of the game, instead of returning

to the locker room to enjoy the team's victory, I simply

asked Dad to drive me home. I think at that moment, I

finally came to terms with my situation. Surgery was the

right answer for me.

My Cardiac Trailblazers

5 – *A Remarkable Second Chance*

On December 12, 1977, I had my second open-heart surgery and was once again blessed with an excellent outcome. A modified Right Blalock-Taussig shunt procedure was performed on me by Dr. Kilman at the Ohio State University Hospital in Columbus. The chosen procedure was modified during the surgery itself due to the small size of my subclavian arteries. Dr. Kilman reported using a Gortex graft as the shunt to connect my right subclavian artery to my right pulmonary artery. The result was to allow more oxygenated blood to alleviate the restriction caused by the previous pulmonary artery banding.

The doctors remarked in their notes that my color improved almost immediately and that there was good blood flow through the shunt. Following me through recovery, doctors Kilman and Hosier commented on the remarkable improvement of both my color and exercise tolerance. From my perspective, I gained an appreciation for knowing the difference between how poorly I felt in December 1977 compared with how well I felt by early 1978. It was truly an astounding improvement and I relished the opportunity for another chance to be normal!

The real test of my recovery came January 26, 1978 with the Blizzard of '78. Almost exactly 6 weeks after the surgery, the blizzard struck in the middle of the night, cutting off our electricity for thirty-six hours and quickly plunging temperatures in the house due to a blown-out cellar window. Dad was stuck in Louisville, Kentucky on a business trip. Mom, my grandfather Ervin and I were stranded at home with no way out due to the snow drifts. Fortunately, Dick was able to walk the two miles from Denison University the night of the storm to join us at home. We survived by blocking off the family room in our house, hanging blankets in the doorways. Our only source of heat was the fireplace which we tended throughout. We were able to keep the single room slightly above freezing while it was near zero with strong winds outside.

While Mom was very worried, I was feeling great and secretly enjoying the challenge the blizzard presented. We were bundled up in heavy clothes and so I probably didn't fully grasp the real danger we were in. For me, this was a huge improvement from how I felt at that football game in October. When the electricity came back on and the danger had passed, I felt a real sense of accomplishment. I was reveling in how much better I felt and anxious to get back on track to my normal life.

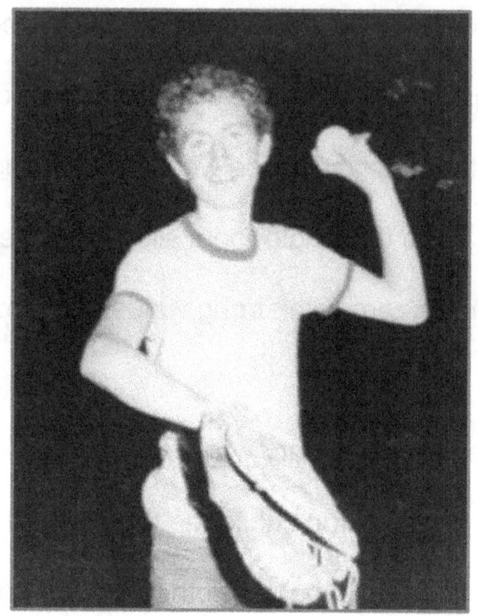

Figure 3 Spring 1978

6 – *What CHD?*

For the remaining two and a half years of high school, my CHD receded into the background. Once I got my strength back, I was again playing pick-up games of football and basketball. I remember being astounded at how much energy I had. Walking 18 holes of golf was relatively easy, although carrying my clubs tested my limits and was very difficult on hilly courses. With that limitation noted, I compromised by using a pull cart and went on to play a lot of golf with family and friends!

In the fall of 1980, I entered Kenyon College. I felt well enough physically to play intramural football and volleyball and was able to keep up with the other players since the games were relaxed and not overly competitive. By sophomore year, I had added basketball and softball to my list of activities. I knew my parents were worried about how I'd adjust to college and so I may not have mentioned the extent of my intramural participation until well after graduation.

I was in pretty good shape in college, though. The Kenyon campus layout required substantial walking to every class, meal and activity. I quickly got used to walking and it really increased my stamina. For the most part, I pushed my CHD to the back of my mind. The only time it was really an issue was following intramural football and basketball games. After pushing myself to my limit and sometimes beyond it during the games, I faced the daunting prospect of climbing "the hill" after each game. Trying to keep up with my friends to get to the dining hall was always a struggle and a gnawing reminder that my CHD was still there. I'm not sure they noticed how I always seemed to stop halfway up the hill to tie my shoe, allowing me to catch my breath. To me the temporary fatigue was well worth it. I absolutely loved participating in

My Cardiac Trailblazers

intramural sports and the feeling of being a part of a team that came with it!

Throughout high school and college, my parents were diligent about scheduling checkups with Dr. Hosier. These occurred every two years and I got used to hearing the report that I was doing well and OK to continue for another two years. By this time, going to Children's Hospital for these visits was increasingly awkward. The equipment was designed for children as was the décor, but I really liked Dr. Hosier and so I put up with it. I had not grasped the reality that there were no adult congenital heart cardiologists in the early 1980s and there was nowhere else I could go to receive the right care. And because I felt so well and couldn't envision my health changing, I didn't really consider what that meant to my future.

After graduating Kenyon in 1984, I went straight into graduate school at Ohio State. I wasn't ready to jump into the work world and was not sure what I wanted to do for a career. I think my parents were relieved that the two-year program would give me time to mature and that I would be sharing an apartment with my brother Dick.   I stayed in decent shape with all the walking required to get from the Ohio State parking lots to my classes.

During winter of my second year of graduate school, I decided to join an intramural basketball team. I remember the first (and last) game I played in that league. It should have been eye opening for me but wasn't. Running the court seemed much harder than I remembered, and I could not keep up with the other players. After running up and down the court a few times, I was thoroughly exhausted. I attributed it to being out of shape, but now I think this was the first indication that my Blalock-Taussig shunt was starting to deteriorate.

My Cardiac Trailblazers

Unwisely, I didn't mention this to anyone and tried not to think about it.

7 – *Nearly Lost to Care*

After completing graduate school in June 1986, I accepted an entry-level position with a cost accounting firm in Richmond, Virginia. My parents were concerned with me moving so far away, but I was determined to go out and establish my own life. I put my CHD out of my mind and moved south without giving much thought to being 500 miles away from my family, friends and the doctor who had supported me for 14 years.

Soon after moving to Virginia, I found a good family practice doctor to provide basic care. He did his best to understand my CHD and was fascinated by it, but I don't think he ever fully grasped it. From a cardiology perspective, I told myself I could always travel back to Ohio for my routine checkups, which I did in October 1986. I mostly felt fine and really didn't give the topic much thought.

For the first year and a half, life in Virginia was good. I was part of a growing business and each new client was a challenge. In the back of my mind, something told me my stamina was decreasing. I thought maybe it was just the high temperatures and humidity in Virginia. The adventure of it all made it easy to push any concerns aside. My cardiac situation was getting incrementally worse, but I ignored it. At this point, I didn't have a local cardiologist and wasn't aware there might be a specialty for adult congenital care for my CHD on the horizon.

By early 1988, the deterioration of my physical stamina was undeniable. The signs were apparent whenever I had to carry anything up the two flights of stairs to my apartment. I started to notice a lot of similarities to my situation in 1977. I was becoming more fatigued and noticeably cyanotic. My normal one-mile walks in Huguenot Park became fewer and shorter and I had less desire to do any kind of exertion.

By April, the situation was becoming difficult and my frustration was growing. Even carrying my briefcase filled with papers was becoming a struggle. I remember going to the park one day with the idea that if I just got into shape, things would get better. I tried to run but couldn't go more than 30 yards before being completely out of breath.   A friend at work convinced me to join a fitness club, but after a few frustrating trips there to lift weights, I knew my situation was dire and I should do something.

8 – Mayo: Yet Another Second Chance

With seemingly nowhere to turn, but knowing denial would not work, fate again smiled on me and a guiding hand sent me in the right direction. After contacting Dr. Hosier and explaining the situation, he referred me to a pediatric cardiologist at the Medical College of Virginia. That doctor was quickly able to determine that my Blalock-Taussig shunt was deteriorating; reducing the volume of blood that could pass through it. I would soon be back in the same situation as 1977. He recommended a catheterization and spoke of probable surgery to replace the shunt.

Now I was facing the prospect of surgery in a strange hospital in Virginia, a new pediatric cardiologist and no local family support. This did not feel like the best situation. Then came a letter from Dr. Hosier. It contained an article about the great work the Mayo Clinic was doing with adult CHD patients using a procedure called the Fontan. By 1988, this procedure had become routine for helping babies and young children with my CHD diagnosis. For them, the Fontan procedure had replaced the pulmonary artery banding technique as the accepted correction a decade earlier. Doctors at the Mayo Clinic were starting to use this same procedure on adults and were having good success. Could I be blessed yet again to have the right doctors with the right surgical solution at the right time to allow me to go on?

My optimism was restored. Although apprehensive about another impending open-heart surgery, I was now mature enough to grasp the reality of the situation. Reflecting on talks with Aunt Joan and Dr. Griffiths eleven years earlier, I was confident I could go through with it this time. Dr. Hosier referred me to the Mayo Clinic in

Rochester, Minnesota. A September appointment was confirmed.

Even though I was now nearly 27 years old, my parents insisted on being there with me every step of the way. After all, they had been through all the other procedures with me and weren't about to be left out of this one. I happily agreed to reassemble this winning team! In early September, we traveled to Mayo.

Mom, Dad and I were all immediately impressed with the efficiency and organization at the Mayo Clinic. All necessary appointments, the catheterization and possible surgery date were set when we got there. Every detail was explained to us prior to each test. Dr. Donald Hagler was my assigned cardiologist. We felt very comfortable with him as he seemed to be cut from the same calm, confident fabric as Doctors Griffiths and Hosier. This put us even more at ease and this time, the situation felt right.

Testing began on Monday, September 5, was finished by Wednesday and to my astonishment, Fontan surgery was scheduled for two days later. On Friday, September 9, 1988, after a seemingly endless day of delays, I was called mid-afternoon into surgery with Dr. Francisco J. Puga at St. Mary's Hospital.   The procedure lasted well into the evening including bypass time of 140 minutes. According to the records, the surgery included interruption of the Blalock-Taussig shunt, resection of the subaortic stenosis and a Modified Fontan operation.

The Fontan procedure was a success. I stayed in the hospital for almost two weeks and then we drove back to Ohio to allow me time to recover and get my strength back. As with my surgery in 1977, I quickly realized how much better I felt and pushed to get back to normal as quickly as I could. In under two months I was back at work in Virginia with renewed energy and stamina. Feeling great again, I had been blessed with yet another "second chance" and was determined to take advantage of it.

9 – More than Ever Hoped For

Within six months and with a renewed sense of purpose, I decided to change my career direction, quit my job, moved back to Ohio. Just two weeks later, I met Theresa Ann O'Connor, the love of my life! I then launched my new career in IT as a programmer. Theresa and I were married June 15, 1991 and were blessed again when we completed our family with the births of our wonderful daughters Ashley in 1994 and Rachel in 1996. Theresa, Ashley and Rachel soon became the core of my CHD support system as they are to this day.

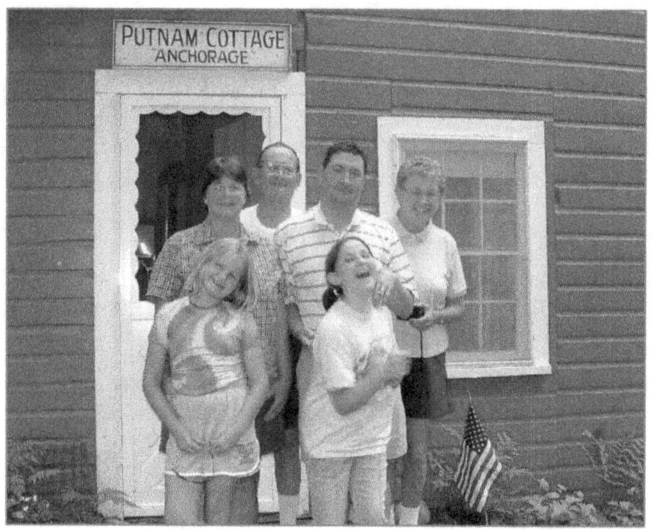

Figure 4 July 2005 at our Camp in Maine

I was living that normal life I had always envisioned, and it became more than I could have ever hoped, despite numerous ongoing challenges of CHD which I have not documented here but inevitably appear and must be faced.

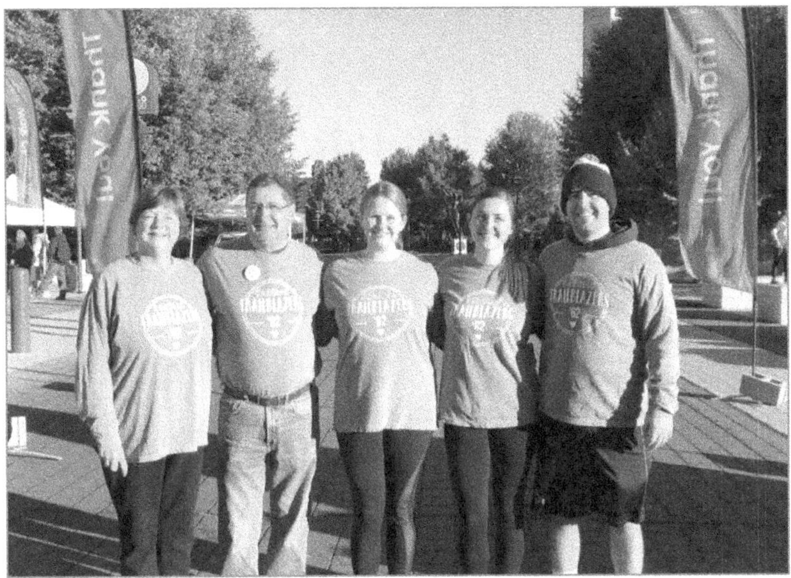

Figure 5 Our 2019 Congenital Heart Walk Team now including Ashley's fiancé Matt Hofacre

Epilogue

Many times, I get caught up in the routine of my normal, everyday life where my CHD is merely an afterthought. I'm mostly pleased with that and I consider my lifelong objective of a normal life to be achieved.   But thirty years provides valuable perspective. Reflecting on my CHD journey today, I acknowledge I really should be more appreciative. Knowing what has benefitted me, given my original diagnosis, I am extremely thankful. I'm also very optimistic for all those CHD children who have and will continue to benefit from the ever-accelerating advancements in medical skill and technology. I'm also exceedingly proud to have been given the opportunity to be a participant in several of these advancements!

I am grateful that my Fontan correction has enabled me to continue for over thirty years now. That surgery ushered in the best years of my life. I will be forever thankful to God, my "Cardiac Trailblazers," my family and friends as well as the incredible advancements in medical science for making these last 30 plus years possible. Because of all these factors, I'm now able to look back on Theresa and I raising and supporting our family, having a successful career and sending Ashley and Rachel out on their life journeys.

Without any one of these factors, none of this would have been possible. For me, living a normal life was the objective. In retrospect, it's been that and so much more than "normal." It is remarkable! At times I reflect on this and find myself thinking: "Not a bad journey for a kid with CHD, originally given just a few months to live! "

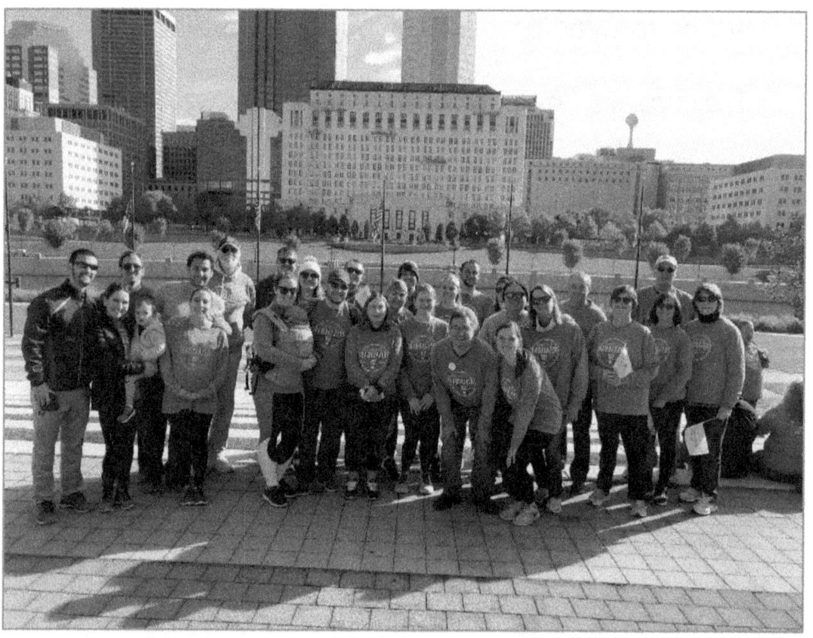

Figure 6 My Cardiac Trailblazers '62 Team 2019, at the Central Ohio Congenital Heart Walk in Columbus

My Cardiac Trailblazers